Table of Contents

INTRODUCTION

Living well with Barrett's esophagus can be a challenging endeavor, but with the right knowledge and lifestyle adjustments, it is entirely possible to lead a fulfilling and healthy life. Barrett's esophagus is a condition in which the lining of the esophagus, the tube that connects the mouth to the stomach, becomes damaged due to chronic acid reflux. While it is a precursor to a more serious condition called esophageal adenocarcinoma, it doesn't always progress to cancer. Managing Barrett's esophagus primarily involves preventing further damage to the esophagus and minimizing the risk of cancer development.

One crucial aspect of living well with Barrett's esophagus is maintaining a diet that is gentle on the esophagus and reduces acid reflux. This often means avoiding trigger foods, such as spicy or acidic foods, caffeine, alcohol, and high-fat meals, which can exacerbate symptoms. Instead, a Barrett's esophagus cookbook can provide valuable guidance on creating meals that are not only delicious but also soothing to the esophagus.

In this cookbook, I will explore a variety of recipes and culinary techniques designed specifically for individuals with Barrett's esophagus. These recipes aim to minimize reflux, discomfort, and irritation while maximizing flavor and nutrition. You will find dishes that are low in acid, easy to digest, and gentle on the sensitive esophageal lining. Additionally, I will incorporate ingredients known for their potential to alleviate symptoms, such as ginger and aloe vera, to create dishes that promote overall well-being.

Throughout this cookbook, you'll discover tips on meal planning, portion control, and eating habits that can contribute to a healthier, more comfortable life with Barrett's esophagus. I understand that dietary restrictions can be challenging, but they need not be limiting. With a little creativity and the right recipes, you can enjoy a wide range of flavorful and satisfying dishes that support your health and well-being.

Remember, living well with Barrett's esophagus is not just about what you eat; it's also about making positive lifestyle choices, managing stress, and seeking regular medical care to monitor your condition. This cookbook is designed to be a valuable resource on your journey to maintaining a balanced and enjoyable diet while minimizing the risk of complications associated with Barrett's esophagus. Let's embark on this culinary adventure together and discover how delicious and fulfilling a Barrett's esophagus-friendly diet can be.

BARRETT'S ESOPHAGUS

Barrett's esophagus is a medical condition that affects the lining of the lower esophagus. It is typically associated with chronic gastroesophageal reflux disease (GERD), a condition in which stomach acid flows back into the esophagus, causing irritation and inflammation over time. In response to this chronic irritation, the normal lining of the esophagus can be replaced by specialized cells that are more similar to those found in the intestines. This change in the lining is known as metaplasia.

KEY POINTS ABOUT BARRETT'S ESOPHAGUS:

- **Precursor to Esophageal Adenocarcinoma:** Barrett's esophagus is a significant concern because it is considered a precursor to esophageal adenocarcinoma, a type of esophageal cancer. Although not everyone with Barrett's esophagus will develop cancer, regular monitoring is recommended to detect any changes early.

• Risk Factors: The primary risk factor for developing Barrett's esophagus is chronic GERD or acid reflux. Other factors, such as obesity and smoking, may also increase the risk.

• Symptoms: Many individuals with Barrett's esophagus may not experience noticeable symptoms. Instead, they often have symptoms related to GERD, such as heartburn, regurgitation, and difficulty swallowing.

• Diagnosis: Diagnosis is typically made through an upper endoscopy, during which a small tissue sample (biopsy) is taken from the esophagus to confirm the presence of specialized cells.

• Management: The primary goal in managing Barrett's esophagus is to control acid reflux and prevent further damage to the esophagus. This may involve lifestyle changes (diet and weight management), medication (proton pump inhibitors), and, in some cases, surgical procedures to repair the lower esophageal sphincter.

- **Monitoring**: Regular follow-up endoscopies are recommended to monitor the condition and detect any precancerous changes or cancerous growth early. This allows for timely intervention if necessary.

BARRETT'S ESOPHAGUS DIET COOKBOOK

MAIN DISH

Chicken and Pea Risotto

Ingredients

- 2 tbsp. mild olive oil or sunflower oil

- 1 onion, cut in half, coarsely grated

- 2 garlic cloves, grated

- 250g/9oz Arborio risotto rice

- 100ml/3½fl oz white wine, dry vermouth or water

- 1 litre/1¾ pints chicken stock cube, made with 1 stock cube

- 250g/9oz cooked leftover chicken, skin removed, cut into small pieces

- 200g/7oz frozen peas

- 75g/2¾oz Grana Padano or other hard Italian-style cheese, finely grated

- 25g/1oz butter

- Freshly ground black pepper

Method

- Heat the oil in a large, non-stick saucepan over a medium heat. Add the onion and garlic and fry for 2-3 minutes, stirring occasionally, until softened and just beginning to colour.

- Add the risotto rice to the pan and stir well for 30-40 seconds, until the oil has coated the grains of rice.

- Pour in half of the wine and allow to bubble for 30-40 seconds, then add all of the stock and bring to the boil, stirring well. Reduce the heat and simmer, uncovered, for 8-10 minutes, stirring frequently, until the rice is almost tender and the risotto is creamy in appearance.

- Stir in the remaining wine, the chicken and the frozen peas, then continue to cook, stirring constantly, for a further 4-5 minutes, or until the chicken and peas are heated through and the rice is tender with a slight bite.

• Remove the pan from the heat, then stir in the butter and cheese. Season with black pepper.

• Cover the pan with a lid and set aside for 5 minutes before serving.

LUNCH

1. Chicken and Vegetable Stir-Fry:

Ingredients:

• Boneless, skinless chicken breast

• Mixed vegetables (e.g., broccoli, bell peppers, carrots)

• Low-sodium soy sauce

• Garlic, minced

• Ginger, grated

Instructions:

• Stir-fry chicken and vegetables in a non-stick pan with a small amount of oil. Add garlic and ginger for flavor.

2. Baked Salmon with Quinoa:

Ingredients:

• Salmon fillet

• Quinoa

• Lemon juice

• Fresh dill

• Olive oil

Instructions:

• Season salmon with lemon juice and dill. Bake until cooked. Serve with cooked quinoa.

3. Turkey and Avocado Wrap:

Ingredients:

- Sliced turkey breast

- Sliced avocado

- Whole wheat tortilla

- Lettuce and tomato

Instructions:

- Assemble turkey, avocado, lettuce, and tomato in a whole wheat tortilla for a flavorful wrap.

4. Mashed Sweet Potatoes:

Ingredients:

- Sweet potatoes

- Low-fat yogurt

- Cinnamon (optional)

Instructions:

• Steam or bake sweet potatoes until soft, mash them, and mix with a dollop of low-fat yogurt.

5. Tuna Salad Lettuce Cups:

Ingredients:

• Canned tuna (in water)

• Greek yogurt

• Celery, finely chopped

• Dill, chopped

• Butter lettuce leaves

Instructions:

• Mix tuna, Greek yogurt, celery, and dill. Serve in lettuce cups.

6. Vegetable Soup:

Ingredients:

• Mixed vegetables (carrots, zucchini, spinach)

• Low-sodium vegetable broth

• Herbs and spices (e.g., basil, oregano)

Instructions:

• Simmer vegetables in vegetable broth with herbs and spices until tender.

7. Grilled Chicken Salad:

Ingredients:

• Grilled chicken breast

• Mixed greens

• Cherry tomatoes

• Cucumber slices

• Balsamic vinaigrette (low-acid)

Instructions:

• Combine grilled chicken, mixed greens, cherry tomatoes, and cucumber. Drizzle with low-acid balsamic vinaigrette.

8. Baked Cod with Steamed Asparagus:

Ingredients:

• Cod fillet

• Asparagus spears

• Lemon zest and juice

• Olive oil

Instructions:

• Season cod with lemon zest and juice. Bake and serve with steamed asparagus.

9. Brown Rice and Lentil Bowl:

Ingredients:

• Cooked brown rice

• Cooked lentils

• Sautéed spinach and mushrooms

• Olive oil and lemon dressing

Instructions:

• Combine brown rice, lentils, sautéed spinach, and mushrooms. Drizzle with olive oil and lemon dressing.

10. Greek Yogurt Parfait:

Ingredients:

• Greek yogurt

• Fresh berries (e.g., strawberries, blueberries)

• Honey (optional)

• Granola (low-fat)

Instructions:

• Layer Greek yogurt, fresh berries, honey, and low-fat granola for a tasty parfait.

11. Spinach and Feta Stuffed Chicken Breast:

Ingredients:

• Chicken breast

• Spinach

• Reduced-fat feta cheese

• Garlic powder

Instructions:

• Stuff chicken breast with spinach and feta, season with garlic powder, and bake until cooked through.

12. Baked Eggplant Parmesan:

Ingredients:

• Sliced eggplant

• Low-acid tomato sauce

• Reduced-fat mozzarella cheese

Instructions:

• Layer eggplant slices with low-acid tomato sauce and reduced-fat mozzarella. Bake until bubbly.

13. Quinoa and Black Bean Salad:

Ingredients:

• Cooked quinoa

• Black beans (canned, rinsed)

• Corn kernels

• Chopped cilantro

• Lime dressing (olive oil, lime juice)

Instructions:

• Mix quinoa, black beans, corn, and cilantro. Drizzle with lime dressing.

14. Mashed Cauliflower:

Ingredients:

• Cauliflower florets

• Low-fat milk or almond milk

• Chopped chives

Instructions:

• Steam cauliflower until tender, mash with low-fat milk, and sprinkle with chives.

15. Roasted Turkey and Veggie Bowl:

Ingredients:

• Sliced roasted turkey

• Roasted vegetables (zucchini, carrots, bell peppers)

• Brown rice

• Low-sodium turkey gravy (optional)

Instructions:

• Assemble turkey, roasted vegetables, and brown rice in a bowl. Add low-sodium turkey gravy if desired.

16. Baked Chicken Tenders with Sweet Potato Fries:

Ingredients:

• Chicken tenders (breaded with whole wheat breadcrumbs)

• Sweet potato fries

• Olive oil

Instructions:

• Bake chicken tenders and sweet potato fries with a drizzle of olive oil until crispy.

17. Quinoa and Avocado Salad:

Ingredients:

• Cooked quinoa

• Sliced avocado

• Cherry tomatoes

• Fresh basil leaves

• Balsamic vinaigrette (low-acid)

Instructions:

• Combine quinoa, avocado, cherry tomatoes, and fresh basil. Drizzle with low-acid balsamic vinaigrette.

18. Butternut Squash Soup:

Ingredients:

• Butternut squash, roasted or steamed

• Low-sodium chicken or vegetable broth

• Nutmeg (optional)

Instructions:

• Blend roasted or steamed butternut squash with low-sodium broth. Season with nutmeg if desired.

19. Tofu and Vegetable Stir-Fry:

Ingredients:

• Extra-firm tofu, cubed

• Mixed vegetables (e.g., broccoli, snap peas, bell peppers)

• Low-sodium teriyaki sauce

Instructions:

• Stir-fry tofu and vegetables in a non-stick pan with low-sodium teriyaki sauce.

20. Lentil and Vegetable Soup:

Ingredients:

• Brown lentils

• Mixed vegetables (carrots, celery, onions)

• Low-sodium vegetable broth

• Herbs and spices (e.g., thyme, rosemary)

Instructions:

• Cook lentils and vegetables in low-sodium vegetable broth with herbs and spices until tender.

DINNER

Baked Herb-Crusted Salmon:

Ingredients:

• Salmon fillet

• Fresh herbs (e.g., parsley, dill, chives)

• Lemon juice

• Olive oil

Instructions:

• Coat salmon with chopped herbs, lemon juice, and a drizzle of olive oil. Bake until cooked through.

2. Grilled Turkey Burger with Sweet Potato Fries:

Ingredients:

• Ground turkey

• Whole wheat burger buns

• Sweet potato fries (baked)

Instructions:

• Grill turkey burgers and serve on whole wheat buns with baked sweet potato fries.

3. Roasted Chicken with Steamed Broccoli and Quinoa:

Ingredients:

• Chicken breast or thigh

• Broccoli florets (steamed)

• Quinoa

• Lemon zest and juice

Instructions:

• Roast chicken with lemon zest and juice. Serve with steamed broccoli and quinoa.

4. Vegetable and Tofu Stir-Fry:

Ingredients:

• Extra-firm tofu

• Mixed vegetables (e.g., bell peppers, snap peas, carrots)

• Low-sodium stir-fry sauce

Instructions:

• Stir-fry tofu and vegetables with low-sodium stir-fry sauce.

5. Spaghetti Squash with Tomato and Basil Sauce:

Ingredients:

• Spaghetti squash

• Tomato and basil sauce (low-acid)

• Fresh basil leaves

Instructions:

• Roast spaghetti squash and serve with low-acid tomato and basil sauce. Garnish with fresh basil.

6. Grilled Shrimp Skewers with Rice Pilaf:

Ingredients:

• Shrimp (peeled and deveined)

• Bell peppers, onions, and zucchini (cut into chunks)

• Rice pilaf

• Lemon juice

Instructions:

• Thread shrimp and vegetables onto skewers, grill, and serve with rice pilaf. Drizzle with lemon juice.

7. Baked Cod with Garlic Butter Sauce:

Ingredients:

• Cod fillet

• Garlic, minced

• Butter (or olive oil)

• Fresh parsley

Instructions:

• Bake cod with garlic and butter (or olive oil). Garnish with fresh parsley.

8. Quinoa and Chickpea Stuffed Bell Peppers:

Ingredients:

• Bell peppers

• Cooked quinoa

• Chickpeas

• Chopped tomatoes

• Herbs and spices (e.g., cumin, paprika)

Instructions:

• Stuff bell peppers with a mixture of cooked quinoa, chickpeas, chopped tomatoes, and herbs and spices. Bake until peppers are tender.

9. Baked Turkey Meatballs with Spaghetti Squash:

Ingredients:

• Ground turkey

• Whole wheat breadcrumbs

• Spaghetti squash

• Low-acid tomato sauce

Instructions:

• Make turkey meatballs with whole wheat breadcrumbs. Serve with roasted spaghetti squash and low-acid tomato sauce.

10. Baked Eggplant and Zucchini Parmesan:

Ingredients:

• Sliced eggplant and zucchini

• Low-acid tomato sauce

• Reduced-fat mozzarella cheese

Instructions:

• Layer sliced eggplant and zucchini with low-acid tomato sauce and reduced-fat mozzarella. Bake until bubbly.

11. Lemon Herb Grilled Chicken:

Ingredients:

• Chicken breast

• Lemon juice and zest

• Fresh herbs (e.g., rosemary, thyme)

• Olive oil

Instructions:

• Marinate chicken in lemon juice, zest, herbs, and olive oil. Grill until cooked through.

12. Lentil and Spinach Soup:

Ingredients:

• Brown or green lentils

• Fresh spinach leaves

• Low-sodium vegetable broth

• Herbs and spices (e.g., coriander, cumin)

Instructions:

• Simmer lentils and spinach in low-sodium vegetable broth with herbs and spices until tender.

13. Baked Butternut Squash Risotto:

Ingredients:

• Butternut squash, roasted and mashed

• Arborio rice

• Low-sodium vegetable broth

• Fresh sage leaves

Instructions:

• Prepare risotto with mashed butternut squash, low-sodium vegetable broth, and fresh sage.

14. Greek Chicken Souvlaki Salad:

Ingredients:

• Grilled chicken skewers

• Greek salad (cucumber, tomato, red onion, olives, feta)

• Tzatziki sauce (low-fat)

Instructions:

• Serve grilled chicken skewers on a bed of Greek salad with a dollop of low-fat tzatziki sauce.

15. Baked Sweet Potatoes with Black Bean Salsa:

Ingredients:

• Sweet potatoes

• Black bean salsa (low-acid)

• Chopped cilantro

Instructions:

• Bake sweet potatoes and top with low-acid black bean salsa. Garnish with chopped cilantro.

16. Lemon Garlic Shrimp and Asparagus:

Ingredients:

• Shrimp (peeled and deveined)

• Asparagus spears

• Lemon juice and zest

• Olive oil

Instructions:

• Sauté shrimp and asparagus in olive oil with lemon juice and zest until cooked.

17. Spinach and Feta Stuffed Portobello Mushrooms:

Ingredients:

• Portobello mushrooms

• Spinach

• Reduced-fat feta cheese

• Garlic powder

Instructions:

• Stuff portobello mushrooms with spinach and reduced-fat feta. Season with garlic powder and bake.

18. Chicken and Vegetable Curry:

Ingredients:

• Chicken breast (cut into cubes)

• Mixed vegetables (e.g., bell peppers, peas, carrots)

• Curry sauce (low-acid)

Instructions:

• Cook chicken and vegetables in low-acid curry sauce.

19. Baked Halibut with Lemon Herb Butter:

Ingredients:

• Halibut fillet

• Lemon juice and zest

• Fresh herbs (e.g., tarragon, chives)

• Butter (or olive oil)

Instructions:

• Bake halibut with lemon juice, zest, fresh herbs, and butter (or olive oil).

20. Turkey and Quinoa Stuffed Bell Peppers:

Ingredients:

• Bell peppers

• Ground turkey

• Cooked quinoa

• Chopped tomatoes

• Herbs and spices (e.g., oregano, basil)

Instructions:

• Stuff bell peppers with a mixture of cooked ground turkey, quinoa, chopped tomatoes, and herbs and spices. Bake until peppers are tender.

Complan Soup

Ingredients

• 1 tin or packet of soup

• 3 heaped dessert spoons natural flavour Complan

Method

• Heat enough soup for one serving, following the instructions on the tin or packet.

• Mix Complan with a little cold water to make a smooth paste.

• Remove soup from heat and slowly stir in the Complan.

Complan Angel Delight

Ingredients

• 1 packet Angel Delight

• 3 heaped dessert spoons natural flavour Complan

• ½ pint cold water

Method

• Mix Complan with a little water to make a thin cream, then add the remaining water.

• Sprinkle in the dessert powder and whisk briskly

Build-Up Milk Jelly

Ingredients

• 1 sachet strawberry Build-Up

• 1 packet strawberry jelly

• ½ pint milk or fortified milk or vanilla Ensure

Method

• Dissolve jelly in a little boiling water and make up to ¾ pint with cold water.

• Mix Build-Up with the milk.

• When jelly is cold but not set, stir slowly into the Build-Up.

• Pour into individual dishes or moulds and leave to set.

• Alternative flavours. Vanilla Build-Up with various jelly flavours, or chocolate.

Build-Up Yogurt

Ingredients

• ½ sachet Build-Up

• 5oz carton natural full-fat yoghurt

Method

• You may find Build-Up too sweet: mixing it with plain yogurt gives it a much sharper flavour.

Ensure instant Soup

Ingredients

• 1 can Ensure

• 1 packet instant soup mix (e.g. Cup-A-Soup)

Method

• Heat Ensure but do not boil, add soup mix, stir well, blend and serve.

Winter Vegetable Soup

Ingredients

• (It makes lots – so freeze half. You will need a blender)

• 500g Potatoes

- 300g Carrots

- 2 large onions

- 4 cloves of garlic

- 1 large leek

- 300g parsnips

- 300g swede

- Small bunch of chopped parsley

- 2 vegetable stock cubes or 2 tbsp.

- bouillon/broth

- Olive Oil

- Salt and Pepper

Method

- Peel and chop the potatoes, parsnips, swede and carrots roughly into 2cm cubes.

- Wash and slice leeks. Peel and chop the onions and garlic.

• Put enough oil in a big pan to cover the bottom and gently fry the vegetables in this order: potatoes, swede, parsnips, carrots, leeks, onions and garlic. With the lid on, cook gently, stirring occasionally until the vegetables are really soft.

• Meanwhile: make the stock. Add the stock cube or bouillon to 2 pints of boiling water. Add to the pan and bring to the boil. Simmer for 5-10 minutes.

• Blend in the pan with a hand-blender or in a food processor.

• Add salt & pepper to taste and serve with the finely chopped parsley.

Cream of Mushroom Soup

Ingredients

• ½lb mushrooms, sliced

• ¾ pint chicken stock

• 1 small onion, chopped

- 1oz butter

- 1oz flour

- ¾ pint milk

- 2 tablespoons cream

- Salt and freshly ground pepper

Method

• Place the mushrooms in a pan with the onion and stock, bring to the boil and simmer for 20 minutes until tender; liquidise.

• Melt butter in a pan, add the flour and cook for 1 minute; gradually blend in the milk and then the prepared mushroom purée and season to taste; bring to the boil and simmer for 5-10 minutes.

• Just before serving stir in the cream.

Yoghurt Cooler

Ingredients

- 5oz carton fruit yoghurt

- ¼ pint milk

Method

- Mix together by hand or in a blender.

- Serve in a glass with straw.

Lemon Water Ice

Ingredients

- Grated rind and juice of one lemon

- 2 oz sugar

- 2 tablespoons of honey

- 1 teaspoon of gelatine

- ½ pint of water

Method

- Heat sugar and water together, allow to boil for five minutes.

• Dissolve gelatine in a little hot water.

• Mix lemon rind, juice and honey into the hot syrup, add gelatine, and stir well.

• Cool, stirring occasionally, then freeze.

• When beginning to set at the edges, whisk with a fork, pour into individual dishes and complete freezing.

Chicken Liver Parfait with French Bread

Ingredients

• 325g unsalted butter, melted and cooled slightly, plus a little extra for greasing

• 500g chickens' liver, trimmed

• 1 garlic clove, crushed

• 2 tbsp. brandy

• Tiny pinch each of ground nutmeg, cloves,

• cinnamon and allspice

• 1 baguette, sliced and toasted, to serve

Method

• Preheat the oven to 110°C/fan 90°C/gas ¼. Grease 8 x 100ml ramekins with melted butter, then set aside.

• Put the liver, garlic, brandy and spices into a food processor. Season with white pepper and 1 teaspoon salt and blend for 1 minute. With the machine still running, add 225g melted butter and blend for a few seconds. Press through a fine sieve into a bowl.

• Divide the mixture among the ramekins and cover with buttered foil. Put in a small roasting tin and pour in hot water to come halfway up the sides of the ramekins.

• Cook for 45 minutes or until just set. Remove from the tin and cool.

• Remove the foil and cover each ramekin with cling film. Chill overnight.

• Slowly melt the remaining butter in a small pan. Remove from the heat set aside for 10 minutes, then pour away the clear butter, leaving just the sediment. Pour a thin film over each parfait and chill until set. Serve with the toast and some onion marmalade.

Wine Recommendation

A luscious pudding win, well-chilled. Try Sauternes or a good value option, Monbazillac.

Vinaigrette Dressing

Ingredients

• 1 rounded teaspoon Maldon sea salt

• 1 clove garlic, peeled

• 1 rounded teaspoon mustard powder

• 1 dessertspoon balsamic vinegar

• 1 dessertspoon sherry vinegar

• 5 tablespoons extra virgin olive oil

• Freshly milled black pepper

Method

• Begin by placing the salt in the mortar and crush it quite coarsely, then add the garlic and, as you begin to crush it and it comes into contact with the salt, it will quickly break down into a purée.

• Next, add the mustard powder and really work it in, giving it about 20 seconds of circular movements to get it thoroughly blended.

• After that, add some freshly milled black pepper. Now add the vinegars and work these in in the same way, then add the oil, switch to a small whisk and give everything a really good, thorough whisking.

• Whisk again before dressing the salad

Eggs Benedict

Ingredients

- 1 quantity Hollandaise Sause

- 6 large, very fresh eggs

- 12 slices of pancetta, grilled until crisp

- 3 English muffins, split in half horizontally

- A little butter

Method

- Pre-heat grill to its highest setting.

- Poach the eggs.

- When the pancetta is cooked, keep it on a warm plate while you lightly toast the split muffins on both sides.

- Now butter the muffins and place them on the baking tray, then top each half with two slices of pancetta.

- Put a poached egg on top of each muffin half and then spoon over the hollandaise, covering the egg (there should be a little over 1 tablespoon of sauce for each egg).

• Now flash the Eggs Benedict under the grill for just 25-30 seconds, as close to the heat as possible, but don't take your eyes off them – they need to be tinged golden and no more.

• This should just glaze the surface of the hollandaise.

• Serve straight away on hot plates.

Avocado Mousse with Prawns and Vinaigrette

Ingredients

• 2 ripe avocados

• ½ oz (10g) powdered gelatine

• 5 fl oz (150ml) hot chicken stock

• 5 fl oz (150ml) soured cream

• 5 fl oz (150ml) mayonnaise

- Juice of half a lemon

- 1 clove garlic, finely chopped

- 3oz (75g) peeled prawns

- Vinaigrette to serve (see Vinaigrette recipe)

- Salt and freshly milled black pepper

Method

- You will also need 8 small ramekins, lightly oiled, a pestle and mortar, a 1 ½ pint (850ml) basin and an electric mixer (or balloon whisk, if you need the exercise).

- To make the avocado mousse, put 3 tablespoons of stock and the gelatine in a bowl and stand it in a pan of simmering water. Stir until the gelatine is dissolved, then pour into the goblet of a liquidiser with the rest of the stock.

- Next, skin and stone the avocados, chop the flesh roughly and add it to the liquidizer (include the darker green part that clings to the skin – this will help the colour). Now add the lemon juice and garlic, and blend until it's completely smooth. Empty the mixture into a bowl and stir in the soured cream and mayonnaise very thoroughly, then season with salt and pepper.

• Spoon the mixture into the lightly oiled ramekins, cover them with cling-film and pop them into the fridge to set. When you're ready to serve, slide a palette knife around the edge of each ramekin and ease the mousse away from the sides. Turn the mousses out on to serving plates, top each one of them with some of the prawns and sprinkle some vinaigrette over each serving. Have plenty of crusty bread ready to go with this.

DESSERT

French Rice Pudding

Ingredients

• 2oz ground rice

- 2oz sugar

- 1 pint fortified milk or milk and vanilla Ensure

- 1 egg

Method

- Heat milk and sugar in a saucepan until almost boiling; sprinkle in the ground rice, stirring well until just boiling.

- Simmer until rice is tender (3-4 minutes) and allow to cool slightly.

- Separate the egg and beat the yolk into the rice. Whisk the egg white and fold into the rice.

- Pour into a greased pie dish and stand it in a shallow pan of hot water.

- Bake at 350°F (180°C, Reg 4) until well risen (about 20 minutes).

Apricot Fool

Ingredients

• 12-16 oz cooked or tinned apricots (or other fruit)

• ½ pint high protein custard (see Sauces)

• Sugar to taste

Method

• Drain the fruit well and sieve or blend to make a thick purée; sweeten to taste.

• Make the custard and whisk with the fruit.

• Pour into individual serving dishes.

• Chill, and serve with cream.

Quick Milk Pudding

Ingredients

• 2oz semolina, ground rice or flaked rice

• 2oz sugar

• 1 pint fortified milk or milk and vanilla Ensure

Method

• Heat milk and sugar until almost boiling.

• Sprinkle in the cereal, stirring well until just boiling.

• Simmer until cooked (3-4 minutes).

• Serve with jam, honey or golden syrup

Baked Egg Custard

Ingredients

• 1 pint of fortified milk

• 3 eggs

• 1oz sugar

• Grated nutmeg (optional)

Method

• Heat the milk until almost boiling.

• Beat the eggs and sugar together and pour the hot milk slowly over them, stirring well.

• Pour into a greased 1 ½ pint baking dish and sprinkle nutmeg on the top.

• Stand the dish in a shallow pan of hot water and bake at 325°F (170°C, Reg 3) until set (30-40 minutes).

• The finely grated rind of an orange can be added to the custard mixture if liked.

Cherry Cheesecake

Ingredients

• 125g digestive biscuits

• 75g soft butter

• 300g cream cheese

• ½ teaspoon lemon juice

• 60g icing sugar

- 1 teaspoon vanilla extract

- 250ml double cream

- 1 x 284g jar St Dalfour Rhapsodie de

- Fruit Black Cherry Spread

Method

- Blitz the biscuits in a food processor until beginning to turn to crumbs, then add the butter and whiz again to make the mixture clump.

- Press this mixture into a 20cm spring-form tin; press a little up the sides to form a slight ridge.

- Beat together the cream cheese, icing sugar, vanilla extract and lemon juice in a bowl until smooth.

- Lightly whip the double cream, and then fold it into the cream cheese mixture.

- Spoon the cheesecake filling on top of the biscuit base and smooth with a spatula.

• Put it in the fridge for 3 hours or overnight.

• When you are ready to serve the cheesecake, un-mould it and spread the black cherry over the top.

Ensure Banana Shake

Ingredients

• 1 banana

• 1 can chilled Ensure

Method

• Peel and slice the banana. Place in blender, add Ensure and blend until smooth.

Milkshake

Ingredients

• 1 cup milk

- 1 packet Build Up or Complan – flavour of your choice

- 1 scoop ice cream

Method

- Blend all ingredients together and serve

Fruit Milkshake

Ingredients

- 1 cup milk

- 1 cup tinned fruit (drained) or fresh fruit

- 1 packet vanilla Build Up, Complan or full cream milk

- 1 teaspoon sugar (optional)

Method

- Liquidise the fruit.

- Add other ingredients.

• Blend and serve.

Banana Smoothie

Ingredients

• ¼ cup of orange juice

• 4 bananas

• 3 scoops of plain ice-cream

• 2 tablespoons of golden syrup

• 3 tablespoons of plain yoghurt

• Lemon juice (optional)

• Sugar (optional)

Method

• Cut the bananas into small pieces and put in the blender.

• Add all the other ingredients.

• Blend on full for 20 seconds.

• Put lemon juice around the rim of the glasses then roll the rim in sugar so it sticks to the lemon juice.

• Serve immediately

Lemon and Melon Burst Smoothie

Ingredients

• ½ cup of diced honeydew melon

• ½ cup of low fat lemon yogurt

• 1 cup frozen green grapes

• 1 tablespoon of chopped fresh mint

• Fresh lemon juice to taste (if preferred)

Method

• Put the honeydew melon and lemon yogurt in a blender.

• Next add the grapes and mint then blend until smooth.

* Taste and add lemon juice if you like.

Yogurt smoothie

Ingredients

* 1 pot full fat yoghurt, flavour of your choice

* 1 banana

* 1 packet Build Up or Complan

* 1 cup milk

* 1 teaspoon sugar (optional)

Method

* Blend all ingredients together

SAUCES

High Protein White Sauce

Ingredients

* 1 pint fortified milk

- 1 ½ oz butter or margarine

- 1 ½ plain flour

Method

- Melt the fat in a saucepan; add the flour and stir well.

- Cook gently for 1-2 minutes and remove from heat.

- Add the milk a little at a time, stirring well to make a smooth sauce.

- Return to heat, stir until sauce boils.

- For a savoury sauce season with salt and pepper; for a sweet sauce add sugar to taste.

- Variations, Cheese sauce; add 2-3oz grated cheese. Parsley Sauce; add 1-2 tablespoons chopped parsley. Egg Sauce; add a chopped hard-boiled egg.

High Protein Custard

Ingredients

• 1 pint fortified milk

• 2 tablespoons custard powder

• 1-2 tablespoons sugar

Method

• Mix sugar and custard powder to a smooth paste with a little cold milk.

• Heat the rest of the milk until just boiling.

• Pour on to the custard powder mixture, stirring well.

• Return to pan, stir until boiling and simmer for 1-2 minutes, stirring all the time.

Chicken-Stuffed Cucumber Soup

Makes 8 servings | 230 calories per serving

Ingredients

Marinade

- 1 egg white

- 1 tablespoon minced fresh ginger

- 2 tablespoons water

- 1 teaspoon salt

- 1 teaspoon tamari (gluten-free soy sauce)

- ¼ teaspoon honey

- 1 tablespoon cornstarch

- Dash of toasted sesame oil

SOUP

- 1 pound ground chicken

- 2 tablespoons cornstarch

- 2 medium cucumbers, peeled, seeded to make a hollow area, and sliced cross wise into 2-inch pieces

- 8 cups chicken stock

- 2 (¼-inch-thick) slices peeled fresh ginger, diced

- 1 teaspoon salt

- 8 shiitake or portobello mushrooms, trimmed and sliced

- 10 sprigs fresh cilantro, chopped, for garnish

- 4 teaspoons sesame oil

Direction

1. Combine all of the marinade ingredients in a bowl.

2. Add the ground chicken, mix well, and let marinate for 5 minutes.

3. Lightly dust the cornstarch inside the cucumber pieces.

4. Stuff each hollowed-out area of cucumber with chicken mixture.

5. Bring the chicken stock to a boil in a soup pot over medium-high heat, then add the sliced ginger and salt.

6. Add the stuffed cucumber pieces, bring back to a boil, then lower the heat to medium-low and gently boil for 10–15 minutes, or until the chicken is cooked through.

7. Add the mushrooms and simmer for 1 minute.

8. Serve hot with the chopped cilantro and a drizzle of sesame oil.

ENTREES

Steamed Mussels & Shrimp Pot

Makes 3–4 servings | 450 calories per serving

Ingredients

• 3–4 tablespoons olive oil

• ½ teaspoon sea salt

- 2 shallots, diced

- 1 bulb fennel (not the green parts), coarsely chopped

- 1–2 large tomatoes, diced

- 1–2 cups chicken stock; enough to cover the bottom of your pot, ½ to 1 inch up the side)

- 4 pounds fresh mussels, scrubbed and debearded

- 1–1½ pounds fresh uncooked shrimp, shell on

- ¼ cup chopped fresh cilantro leaves, for garnish

Direction

1. Place your biggest stockpot with a lid (one that will hold all of the ingredients) over medium-high heat and add the olive oil. Then add the salt, shallots, and fennel. Sauté until soft.

2. Add the tomato and continue to cook.

3. Add the chicken stock and bring to a boil over high heat.

4. When the stock is boiling, add the mussels and shrimp and cover.

5. Every 2–3 minutes, with a large serving utensil, move the mussels and shrimp about so that the bottom ones come to the top.

6. When all of the mussels have opened (discard any that haven't), after about 10–12 minutes of steaming, garnish with cilantro and serve in big bowls.

Four-Star Marinated Smoked Tempeh

Makes 4 servings | 275 calories per serving

Ingredients

- 2 tablespoons tamari (gluten-free soy sauce)

- 1 tablespoon sesame oil

- 1 tablespoon mirin

- 1 tablespoon maple syrup

• 2 tablespoons seaweed-mushroom stock

• 1 pound tempeh (usually this will be two ½-pound packages)

• Apple wood or cherry wood, for smoking

1. Mix together all of the ingredients (except the tempeh and apple wood) in a bowl. Add the tempeh and let marinate for 1 hour.

2. Smoke over apple wood or cherry wood for about 15 minutes, or until browned and aromatic.

Grilled Pork with Savory, Cardamom & Cumin

Makes 8–10 servings | 190 calories per serving

Ingredients

• ¼ cup olive oil

• 1–2 pork tenderloins

• 1–2 teaspoons sea salt

• Savory, ground

• Cardamom, ground

• Cumin, ground

Direction

1. Put the oil on the bottom of a large dish and add the pork tenderloins.

2. With a fork, turn the pork so that it gets lightly coated with the oil; add the salt while turning.

3. Next, sprinkle the three spices liberally on the pork, on at least two sides.

4. Cover tightly with plastic wrap and refrigerate. This meat can stay in the refrigerator for up to 2 days.

5. Preheat the grill on high and when hot, sear the tenderloins for 3–5 minutes on each side.

6. Remove the pork from the grill, cover with foil, and let rest about 5 minutes.

7. Turn down the heat to medium. (If your grill has a temperature gauge, you sear at about 700°F and then cook over medium at 300–400°F.)

8. When the grill is ready, put the pork back on the grill for 20–30 minutes, turning once or twice.

9. When done, place on a cutting board for a few minutes before cutting into ½-inch slices.

Pumpkin Gnocchi with Pistachio Sauce

Makes 4 servings | 380 calories per serving

Ingredients

Gnocchi

• 1 cup roasted pumpkin purée

• 1 teaspoon sea salt

• ¼ teaspoon ground nutmeg

• 1 cup semolina flour

Sauce

- 1 cup raw pistachios

- 1 teaspoon sea salt

- 2 cups soymilk

- 20 fresh sage leaves (preferably with stems attached)

- ½ teaspoon freshly grated nutmeg

Directions

for the gnocchi

1. Combine the pumpkin with the salt and nutmeg and mix well. Slowly incorporate the flour until you have a dough. The less flour you add, the lighter the gnocchi will be.

2. Let the dough rest, covered or wrapped, for a half hour.

3. Divide the dough into 4 equal-size portions.

4. Roll out each portion into 1-inch-diameter logs of dough, flouring lightly as needed.

5. Cut the logs into ¾-inch-long pieces to create the gnocchi.

6. Drop the gnocchi in boiling water. When they float, they are finished. Remove from the water, drain, and sauce immediately. Do NOT make in advance; make them as you are ready to serve them.

Directions for the sauce

1. In a cast-iron skillet over medium-low heat, toast the pistachios, stirring constantly until they smell aromatic. Remove from the heat and place in a blender with the salt and soymilk. Blend until smooth.

2. Transfer the pistachio purée into a saucepan and place over low heat.

3. Add the sage leaves and, stirring regularly, bring to a simmer. Cook, stirring, until the sauce thickens slightly.

4. Add the nutmeg, remove the sage leaves, and serve the sauce with the gnocchi.

Turkey & Mushrooms with Rice

Makes 6 servings | 445 calories per serving

Ingredients

- 6 dried shiitake mushrooms

- 3 tablespoons olive oil

- 1 tablespoon minced fresh ginger

- 1 pound ground turkey

- ½ cup rice wine

- ½ cup tamari (gluten-free soy sauce)

- 2 cups water

- 1 teaspoon sugar

- ½ teaspoon Chinese spice blend

- 1 star anise

• Cooked rice, for serving

• Chopped fresh cilantro, for garnish

• Julienned carrots, for garnish

• Bean sprouts, for garnish

Direction

1. In warm water, soak the mushrooms until soft. Rinse the mushrooms and pat dry. Remove the stems and thinly slice the caps.

2. Heat the oil in a pan over medium-high heat. Add the ginger and sauté for 1 minute. Add the mushrooms and turkey and sauté until the turkey is browned.

3. Add the wine, tamari, water, sugar, Chinese spice blend, and star anise. Bring to a boil, then lower the heat to simmer for 45 minutes.

4. Remove the star anise and discard. Serve over rice and garnish with cilantro, carrots, and bean sprouts.

One-Pot Ginger Chicken Rice

Makes 4 servings | 675 calories per serving

Ingredients

• Marinated chicken

• ⅛ teaspoon salt

• 2 tablespoons tamari (gluten-free soy sauce)

• 2 tablespoons olive oil

• 2 tablespoons rice wine

• 4 chicken breasts

• 6 dried shiitake or portobello mushrooms

• 3 tablespoons olive oil

• 12 (⅛-inch-thick) slices peeled fresh ginger

• 2 cups uncooked jasmine or other long grain rice

1½ cups chicken stock

• ¼ cup rice wine (preferably shaoshing

• Sea salt to taste

- 1–2 tablespoons tamari (gluten-free soy sauce)

- Few dashes of sesame oil

- Chopped fresh cilantro, for garnish

Direction

1. For the marinated chicken, mix the salt, tamari, olive oil, and rice wine in a large bowl. Add the chicken breasts and marinate the chicken for 30 minutes in the refrigerator. Drain and set aside the chicken (discard the marinade).

2. In warm water, soak the mushrooms until soft. Rinse the mushrooms and pat dry. Remove the stems and thinly slice the caps.

3. Heat the oil in a pan over medium-high heat and sauté the ginger until fragrant for 1 minute.

4. Add the rice and mix well to coat with oil.

5. Add the chicken stock, rice wine, and salt to taste and mix well.

6. Transfer to a rice cooker and place the chicken breasts and mushrooms on top. Cook the rice according to the manufacturer's instructions. (Alternatively, if you don't have a rice cooker, cook in a pot on the stovetop for at least 20–25 minutes.)

7. Once the rice and chicken are cooked, let stand for 10 minutes, covered.

8. Meanwhile, mix the tamari and sesame oil in a serving bowl.

9. Garnish the rice and chicken with cilantro and serve with the sauce.

Ginger Tempeh

Makes 4 servings | 180 calories per serving

Ingredients

• 2 teaspoons cornstarch, potato starch, or kudzu ½ cup vegetable stock

• ½ pound tempeh, cut into ½-inch strips

- 2 tablespoons tamari (gluten-free soy sauce)

- 1 tablespoon shaoshing wine, MMGF or dry sherry

- 1 tablespoon mirin

- 1 tablespoon grapeseed oil

- 2 tablespoons chopped fresh ginger

- 1 small head broccoli, cut into small florets

- 2 tablespoons chopped fresh cilantro or basil, for garnish

- Cooked brown rice, for serving

Direction

1. Preheat the oven to 400°F.

2. Dissolve the cornstarch in the stock and set aside.

3. Place the tempeh on an oiled baking sheet and bake for 20 minutes, or until lightly browned. Set aside.

4. In a bowl, mix the tamari, shaoshing, and mirin and set aside.

5. In a hot wok or frying pan over medium-high heat, add the grapeseed oil.

6. Add the ginger and stir-fry for 30 seconds.

7. Add the broccoli and stir-fry for 3 minutes, or until the vegetable is bright green and slightly soft.

8. Add the tamari mixture and stir-fry for 10 more seconds.

9. Add the dissolved cornstarch and stock and stir-fry for 30 seconds, until it bubbles and thickens.

10. Add the tempeh and stir to coat, cooking until warmed through.

11. Garnish with the cilantro and serve with brown rice.

Tuscan-Style White Pork with Rosemary

Makes 6 servings | 285 calories per serving

Ingredients

- 2 small- to medium-size pork tenderloins

- 1 teaspoon sea salt

- 2–3 tablespoons olive oil

- 1 large bunch fresh rosemary, or 2 handfuls

- 1–1½ quarts low-fat milk

Direction

1. Cut each of the pork tenderloins into three pieces and salt all sides.

2. Heat the oil in a soup pot over medium-high and brown the 6 pork pieces.

3. When the pork pieces are browned, lower the heat to medium and add the rosemary.

4. Cover the rosemary and the meat with milk; this will take about a quart, possibly more.

5. Bring to a slow bubbling boil and cook for 45 minutes.

6. Remove the meat and slice, serving each portion with some of the intact rosemary stems.

Tempeh Marsala

Makes 4 servings | 340 calories per serving

Ingredients

Tempeh

• Bowl one: ½ cup white flour mixed with ¼ teaspoon salt

• Bowl two: ½ cup soymilk mixed with ¼ teaspoon salt

• Bowl three: ½ cup cornmeal mixed with ½ teaspoon salt, ½ teaspoon dried oregano, ½ teaspoon dried rosemary, ½ teaspoon dried thyme, and 2 tablespoons nutritional yeast

• 1 pound tempeh, cut into 8 equal-size cutlets

Marsala

- 2 tablespoons olive oil

- ¼ pound cremini mushrooms, thinly sliced

- 1 cup fresh shelled peas

- 1 teaspoon dried oregano

- 1½ teaspoons sea salt

- ½ cup Marsala wine

- ½ teaspoon black pepper (optional)

- ¼ cup chopped fresh basil

Directions

for the Tempeh

1. Preheat the oven to 425°F.

2. Place the 3 bowls in order in a row.

3. Dip a tempeh cutlet once in the flour (bowl one), flip, and dip the other side.

4. Now dip the same cutlet in the soymilk mixture (bowl two), coating both sides, and then dip it in the cornmeal mixture (bowl three), coating both sides.

5. Place the breaded tempeh on a baking sheet lightly coated with oil and repeat with the remaining cutlets.

6. Bake for 30 minutes, or until crisp. (Alternatively, deep-fry until golden brown.)

Directions for the Marsala

1. In a frying pan, heat up the olive oil.

2. Add the mushrooms, peas, oregano, and salt and cook for 5 minutes.

3. Add the Marsala wine, cover, and cook for another 5 minutes, until the alcohol evaporates.

4. Pour over the cutlets.

5. Season with salt and pepper and garnish with basil.

Tofu Cutlets

Makes 4 servings | 160 calories per serving

Ingredients

• 1 pound firm tofu, cut into ½-inch-thick slabs

• ¼ cup cornmeal

• ¼ cup nutritional yeast

• 1 teaspoon sea salt

• 2 tablespoons dried herbs (combination of marjoram, oregano, thyme, basil, sage, rosemary)

• ⅓ cup soymilk or almond milk

• 2 tablespoons olive oil

Direction

1. Preheat the oven to 400°F.

2. Press the tofu by placing the slabs on a towel. Cover with another towel and place a cutting board on the top towel. Place a can or something heavy on the board and let sit for 15 minutes.

3. In a bowl, combine the cornmeal, nutritional yeast, salt, and herbs. Pour the soymilk into a separate bowl.

4. Oil a baking sheet with the olive oil.

5. Dip each piece of tofu in the soymilk and then in the herb-cornmeal mixture, thoroughly coating all sides of each.

6. Place each crusted piece of tofu on the baking sheet, not letting the pieces touch.

7. Bake for 30 minutes, or until nice and crispy.

Basil Chicken

Makes 6 servings | 325 calories per serving

Ingredients

• ¼ cup sesame oil or extra-virgin olive oil

• 10 (⅛-inch-thick) slices peeled fresh ginger

- 2 pounds chicken breast, chopped into bite-size chunks 1 cup rice wine preferably shaoshing, or dry sherry)

- 1 cup tamari (gluten-free soy sauce)

- 2 whole star anise, or 1 tablespoon aniseed

- 1 tablespoon honey

- 1 bunch fresh basil, chopped

- Steamed white rice, for serving

Direction

1. Heat the oil in a pan over medium-high heat, then add the ginger and cook until fragrant, about 1 minute.

2. Add the chicken pieces and brown for 1–2 minutes.

3. Add the rice wine, tamari, star anise, and honey and bring to a boil, then reduce the heat to a simmer and cook for 15 minutes, or until the chicken is cooked through.

4. Stir in the basil and remove from the heat. Serve over rice.

Poached Halibut with Prosciutto

Makes 4 servings | 385 calories per serving

Ingredients

• 1 pound halibut, cut into 4 equal-size pieces

• ½ teaspoon salt

• ½ teaspoon rice wine

• 5 dried shiitake mushrooms

• ¼ cup olive oil

• 4 (⅛-inch-thick) slices peeled fresh ginger

• 10 thin slices prosciutto, chopped

• 10 slices canned bamboo shoots

• 1 cup chicken stock

- 2–4 tablespoons chopped fresh cilantro, for garnish

Direction

1. Marinate the halibut in the salt and rice wine for 10 minutes.

2. Soak the mushrooms in warm water until soft. Rinse the mushrooms and pat dry. Remove the stems and thinly slice the caps.

3. Heat the oil in a pan over medium-high heat, then add the ginger and sauté for 1 minute.

4. Add the mushrooms, prosciutto, and bamboo shoots and sauté for 1 minute.

5. Add the halibut and chicken stock and cover the pan.

6. Poach until the fish is cooked through (poach 10–15 minutes per 1 inch of thickness).

7. Top with cilantro and serve.

Turkey Burger Salad with Black Olives & Avocado

Makes 4 servings | 275 calories per serving

Ingredients

• 1 pound ground turkey (preferably 93% lean/7% fat, as 99% lean can be too dry), formed into 4 patties

• ½ teaspoon sea salt

• 2 heads romaine lettuce, washed and cut or torn into 2- to 3-inch pieces

• 1 medium-size can of small, pitted black olives

• 2 tablespoons extra-virgin olive oil

• 1 teaspoon balsamic vinegar

• 1 avocado, peeled and sliced

Direction

1. Season the turkey patties with the salt and cook on the grill or on the stovetop in a covered frying

pan, over medium to medium-high heat for 4–5 minutes per side.

2. After cooking, put the burgers aside until cool enough to break into bite-size pieces.

3. Place the lettuce, olives, oil, and vinegar in a large salad bowl and toss.

4. Finally, add the burger pieces and avocado slices on top.

Gluten-Free Pasta with Shrimp & Zucchini

Makes 6 servings | 460 calories per serving

Ingredients

• 1 pound gluten-free white-rice spaghetti

• 3–4 medium-size zucchinis, halved lengthwise and then sliced into ¼-inch half-moons

• ½ teaspoon sea salt

• 4 tablespoons olive oil

• 1½–2 pounds shrimp (fresh or frozen, uncooked or cooked), peeled and deveined

• ¾ cup chopped fresh basil leaves, stems removed

Direction

1. Get all of the ingredients ready at the start, because the sauce will take about the same time as the pasta to cook. If the shrimp are frozen, defrost them in cold water and then dry them.

2. Put a large pasta pot filled two-thirds with water over high heat.

3. When the water comes to a vigorous, rolling boil, put the pasta in.

4. Start the sauce when the pasta goes into the boiling water.

5. Salt the zucchini. In a large saucepan over high heat, place half of the olive oil and then add the zucchini. Brown the zucchini slices, turning them with a spatula; try not to "boil" them, which is why a big pan and high heat is best.

6. When the zucchini are almost done, add the shrimp. If they are raw, add more of the olive oil, if needed, then add the basil. Cook until heated through.

7. When the pasta is done, drain and serve in individual bowls.

8. Top with the shrimp and zucchini.

Poached Arctic Char with Dill

Makes 2–4 servings | 210 calories per serving

Ingredients

• 1 pound Arctic char, skin on

• 1–2 teaspoons olive oil

• 1 teaspoon sea salt

• 1 cup chicken or vegetable stock

• 2 teaspoons minced fresh dill, stems removed

Direction

1. Cut the fish in half so that it will fit neatly in your pan, or you may cut it into individual servings.

2. Cover both sides of the fish lightly with the olive oil and then the salt.

3. Heat a shallow pan over medium-high heat, and then add the fish skin-side up.

4. Sauté for 2–3 minutes, until there is some sizzle.

5. Add the chicken stock and half of the dill.

6. When the stock is boiling lightly and steaming, cover the pan with a lid or foil. (If the steaming around the edges of the pan is excessive, lower the heat slightly.)

7. Cook for 12–18 minutes, until the fish skin peels off very easily; that's how you know it is done.

8. Plate and garnish with the rest of the fresh dill.

DESSERTS

Watermelon Sorbet

Makes 4 servings | 15 calories per serving

Ingredients

• 4 cups watermelon purée

• 1 tablespoon lemon zest

Direction

1. Combine the watermelon purée and lemon zest and freeze in an ice cream maker according to the manufacturer's instructions.

Ginger-Carrot Ice Pop

Makes 2 servings | 160 calories per serving

Ingredients

• 2 tablespoons agave

• 2 cups fresh carrot juice

• 2 teaspoons fresh ginger juice

Direction

1. Mix all of the ingredients together and pour into an ice pop mold. Insert sticks and freeze until set.

Cucumber Cooler

Makes 4 servings | 20 calories per serving

Ingredients

• 2 cucumbers (preferably Japanese or Persian), peeled

• 4 quarts water

Direction

1. Purée the cucumbers in a blender with a little of the water until smooth.

2. Combine the purée with the rest of the water.

3. Pour over ice and serve.

Cucumber Sorbet

Makes 4 servings | 50 calories per serving

Ingredients

• 2 pounds cucumbers (preferably Japanese or Persian), peeled

• 1 cup water

• 1 teaspoon lemon zest

• 2 tablespoons maple syrup (optional; this works without any sweetener)

Direction

1. Place all of the ingredients in a blender and purée until smooth.

2. Transfer purée to an ice cream maker and churn until frozen according to manufacturer's instructions.

Kick-Ass Carrot Cookies

Makes 3 dozen cookies | 65 calories per cookie

Ingredients

• 1 cup rolled oats

• 1 cup white flour

• 1 teaspoon ground cinnamon

• 1 teaspoon baking powder

• ½ teaspoon baking soda

• ¼ teaspoon salt

• ½ cup maple syrup

• ½ cup grapeseed oil

• 1 cup grated carrot

• ½ cup dried cherries

Direction

1. Preheat the oven to 375°F.

2. In one bowl, combine the oats, flour, cinnamon, baking powder, baking soda, and salt.

3. In a separate bowl, whisk together the syrup and oil.

4. Add the carrots and dried cherries to the wet mixture and mix well.

5. Pour the wet mixture over the dry mixture and gently combine. Do NOT overmix, or the cookies will be rubbery.

6. Drop 1-teaspoon portions of the mixture on a grapeseed-oiled baking sheet, 2 inches apart. (These cookies only bake well if they are small.)

7. Bake for 10 minutes. Be careful not to overcook, as they burn easily.

Seared Watermelon with Feta & Prosciutto

Makes 2 servings | 75 calories per serving

Ingredients

- 8 (½-inch by ½-inch by 2–3-inch-long) rectangular solids (like square logs), cut from the heart of half a watermelon, avoiding seeds

- 4 thin slices prosciutto

- 2 teaspoons crumbled feta cheese

Direction

1. Place a medium-size frying pan over high heat.

2. When the pan is quite hot, spray it with nonstick cooking spray and place four of the watermelon logs in the frying pan.

3. Turn the logs to sear each of the four sides. If the pan is hot enough, it is about 30 seconds per side. (You want them just to sear a bit, no more.)

4. When the first four watermelon logs have a smidge of black on all sides, remove from the heat and set aside.

5. Repeat the same procedure with the remaining four watermelon logs.

6. To plate, neatly place two pieces of prosciutto on each 8-inch plate and then stack four watermelon logs (two on top of two) per serving on the prosciutto.

7. Garnish each watermelon tower with a teaspoon of feta.

Poached Pears with Tea & Vanilla

Makes 4 servings | 163 calories per serving

Ingredients

- 1 quart water

- 2 vanilla beans, split in half

- 3 cardamom pods

- 1 cinnamon stick

- 2 cloves

- ½ cup maple syrup

• 2 tablespoons jasmine tea leaves, or 4 jasmine tea bags (oolong can be substituted)

• 2 large pears, halved and cored

Direction

1. Bring the water to a boil.

2. Add the vanilla, cardamom, cinnamon, cloves, syrup, and tea.

3. Cover, remove from the heat, and let sit for 10 minutes. Remove the tea (if you have not used tea bags, strain to remove the loose tea leaves).

4. Bring back to a simmer.

5. Add the pears, cover, and cook over low heat for 20 minutes.

Banana Pistachio Ice Cream

Makes 8 servings | 150 calories per serving

Ingredients

- ½ cup raw pistachios

- 2 cups water

- ½ cup maple syrup

- 4 ripe bananas

- ½ teaspoon ground cinnamon

Direction

1. Place all of the ingredients in a blender and purée until totally smooth.

2. Transfer the purée to an ice cream maker and churn until frozen according to the manufacturer's instructions.

Caramelized Bananas

Makes 4 servings | 110 calories per serving

Ingredients

- ¼ cup palm sugar

- ¼ cup water

- 2 bananas, halved lengthwise

Direction

1. In a small frying pan over medium-low heat, combine the sugar and water, stirring until the sugar dissolves.

2. Add the bananas, cook for 5 minutes, and then turn over and cook another 5 minutes.

Natural Fruit Mold

Makes 4 servings | 70 calories per serving

Ingredients

- 2 cups water

- 1 cup fresh blueberry juice

- 2 teaspoons kanten (agar) powder

- Fresh seasonal fruit, sliced

• Seasonal berries

Direction

1. In a saucepan, heat up the water and juice, then add the kanten powder and stir constantly with a whisk to dissolve.

2. Bring the mixture to a boil, lower the heat, and cook, stirring constantly, for 3 minutes.

3. Pour the kanten mixture into a 9 x 13-inch glass baking dish.

4. Decorate with fresh fruit slices and berries.

5. Let set for 2 hours, then chill before serving.

Shaved Fruit Ice

Makes 4 servings | 120 calories per serving

Ingredients

• 4 cups crushed ice

• 4 tablespoons honey

• 4 tablespoons vanilla almond milk

• 2 cups diced seasonal fruits

Direction

1. Divide the crushed ice equally into four serving cups.

2. Drizzle 1 tablespoon honey and 1 tablespoon almond milk over each ice cup.

3. Top each with ½ cup diced fruits.

CONCLUSION

Living well with Barrett's esophagus is a journey that requires careful attention to your dietary choices and overall lifestyle. While this condition presents challenges related to acid reflux and the risk of esophageal cancer, it is entirely possible to lead a fulfilling and healthy life with the right approach. The "Living Well with Barrett's Esophagus: A Cookbook" serves as a valuable resource for individuals with this condition, offering recipes and guidance to help you maintain a balanced and enjoyable diet.

Throughout this cookbook, I've explored a range of recipes tailored to be gentle on the esophagus, minimizing irritation and discomfort. These recipes incorporate ingredients known for their potential to alleviate symptoms and promote overall well-being. From chicken and vegetable stir-fry to quinoa and chickpea stuffed bell peppers, there are numerous flavorful and nutritious options to explore.

However, living well with Barrett's esophagus extends beyond the kitchen. It involves making positive lifestyle changes, including managing stress, maintaining a healthy weight, and seeking regular medical care to monitor your condition. Staying informed about your specific dietary triggers and sensitivities is crucial, as individual experiences can vary significantly.

By following the recommendations in this cookbook and working closely with healthcare professionals or dietitians, you can empower yourself to make informed choices that support your health and minimize the risk of complications associated with Barrett's esophagus. Remember that while certain foods and habits should be avoided, there are still plenty of delicious and satisfying options to enjoy.

In essence, living well with Barrett's esophagus is about finding balance, making informed choices, and embracing a lifestyle that prioritizes your well-being. With dedication and the right resources, you can take control of your health and savor the joy of delicious, Barrett's esophagus-friendly meals while reducing the risks associated with this condition.